3S AND OUR HEALTH

A SHORT GUIDE TO A REWARDING LIFE

RAGHURAJ RAJENDRAN

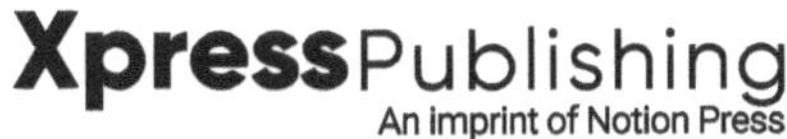

Xpress Publishing

An imprint of Notion Press

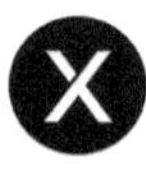

XpressPublishing
An imprint of Notion Press

Old No. 38, New No. 6
McNichols Road, Chetpet
Chennai - 600 031

First Published by Notion Press 2019
Copyright © Raghuraj Rajendran 2019
All Rights Reserved.

ISBN 978-1-64760-092-1

To you

Contents

Foreword

This book tries to tell you something. However, it is not to sell you anything- not even this book. With love for environment in mind, kindly sign on this copy to someone you care for. The contents will always be available for reference on www.3Sandourhealth.org.

Preface

I want this book to be short and straight-forward. It should be able to tell the reader in a crisp manner what is the suggested course of action. For the more curious reader, it needs to clarify the reasoning and references behind what is being suggested for the three objectives – weight management, sleeping well and having good energy levels throughout the day!

I claim no expertise. I only claim experience. I am not a doctor, dietician or a professional fitness expert. This disqualification is also my qualification, as I do not seek to sell you anything but a change in lifestyle at the end of this book.

It is my privilege to assign part of the proceeds of this book towards me to the Social Health One Health Movement. I thank SHOHM for kindly accepting my offer to receive the same. This organisation is a band of volunteers seeking to spread the message of healthy living for the whole of the society. This also helps me find fresh vigour to publish and publicise this book, as I feel I contribute to the cause that is espoused by the organisation.

This book seeks to document my journey in search of a better life. The first bit of publishing in this regard was done on the Facebook and Twitter. Subsequently, these articles have been carried in major journals like The Week, Pioneer and Outlook. In case you prefer a more readable introduction to the concept, I suggest you start with these articles. They are at chapters 10, 11 and 12.

From the contents section, you would notice that the book appears to set out some rules for daily life. A word on this is necessary here. Forget about the rules. Every human body is unique and it would not be wise to set forth rules for each of us to follow as a mandate. It is more important to understand the principle which leads to the rule. Then, if one appreciates the principle, every individual should be able to make an earnest effort to create and calibrate one's own rule to achieve the values espoused.

In my short stint in the Lal Bahadur Shastri National Academy of Administration, officer trainees often came to me for counselling regarding one rule or the other in the academy. There again, I would implore them to go to the first principles and figure out why the rule was imposed. Very often we make the mistake of pronouncing rules without clarifying the linkage between rules and first principles. Conscious individuals should be cautious about this. In this book too, forget the rules; but do look for the logic behind the rules. Then - *atma deepo bhava* !

New Delhi

Raghuraj Rajendran

22.11.2019

Acknowledgements

The book bears its author's name. The author bears a debt to many who, in some way or the other, contributes to the book. I should begin by saying that there would always be some individuals left out when I am acknowledging my debt. My apologies upfront for that!

I thank Dr. Jagannath Dixit for his unwavering support.His work is critical to what is mentioned in the book.Dr Robert Lustig and Dr Suhas Kshirsagar, both of whom I have not met, have left deep impressions on me which is reflected in this book

I thank Shri Dharmendra Pradhan for being supportive and motivating in my efforts. I have been lucky to have Dr. Sanjeev Chopra,Director LBSNAA as my mentor and guide. I take this opportunity to thank him and my other senior colleagues who have always been so encouraging! Shri N Baijendra Kumar, CMD, NMDC, Shri Manoj Jhalani, Ministry of Health, Shri Manoj Ahuja, Special Director, LBSNAA are among them, but this is certainly not the whole list.

I thank Dr. P K Sasidharan for going through the manuscript and suggesting edits.

I thank my colleagues- Jatin, Ankur, Pratyush, Deepak, Yogender, Gora ji and the entire team for being so helpful with my work.

I thank Notion Press for providing a platform where one can publish and still sleep with conscience intact!

I thank my father, who was so enthusiastic to follow me and lead me at the same time.One of the best moments in my life was when he made a call to me to tell that he lost eight kilos and felt more energetic after he followed the regimen. I thank my mother for loving me and believing in me even when she would not believe me! My brother, I am in your arms!

Gowri would complain if I don't mention her name. So would Alli and Appu!But then,it is only a statement of the fact that they are my love.They are my strength. They are my pride. Without them there would be no me, not to speak of the book!

CHAPTER ONE

INTRODUCTION

Introduction

The suggestion is simply this.
 Avoid 3S: Sugar, Snacks, Supper
 Adopt 3S: Sports, Sangeet[1], Sleep

I proceed to elaborate

This book is not about adding years to your life. It is about adding life to your years. If you want the maximum out of your time, read on to get one perspective. The next twenty minutes might change your life!

Many of us struggle to keep our weight in control. We run the risk of becoming diabetic or are already declared diabetic. Some of us feel less than energetic as we move through our day. Some feel that sleep is too short and shallow and detest being alarmed into wakefulness. If you are looking for some tips regarding what to do in this regard, this book has a set of suggestions. They are

1. Avoid refined sugar and sweets.
2. Have your dinner (last meal of the day) before it is dark (1800 hrs).
3. Avoid morning tea before workout.
4. Avoid snacks: Move first to three meals a day- say at 0900, 1300, 1800 hrs.
5. Move to low glycaemic index food (Sprouts, Fruits, Nuts) – Be a natureatarian[2].

6. Move to 2 meals a day.
7. Workout everyday in the morning.

Each of these steps have a definite reasoning behind it. It would be easier to suggest that you should follow this course because religion or some saint suggests so. You would immediately notice that some of the tips are well recognised religious tenets. Traditional wisdom in this regard has been handed down the generations. But the reasoning behind the steps is often lost in transition. In the modern age where information and misinformation is in everyone's finger tips, tenets are not tenacious enough if they are not explained with their reasons. In this book, after starting with the To Do, we proceed to elaborate why.

<u>Notes For the chapter</u>

[1]Sangeet is Hindi/Sanskrit for Music.

[2]This is a high sounding word coined to indicate that one should eat foods which are least processed by homo sapiens.

AVOID SUGAR AND SWEETS!

Avoid sugar and sweets !

If there is to be only one takeaway from this book, this be it. Avoid Sugar! Devoid of this toxin, you will probably set yourself on a course all by yourself and achieve the required end state.

But why this blanket ban on sugar? Here, I suggest you some references. You could pause reading this book and type out 'That Sugar Film' on Google or Youtube. You will find some trailers in the video section and chances are that you will also find the full movie which is about an hour and a half. Watch it ! I watched it and it changed my way of looking at life and my life.

When I saw this movie for the first time, I was struggling to keep faith in the two meals a day diet suggested by Dr. Jagannath Dixit. To achieve intermittent fasting, my plan was to have breakfast and a late lunch. I was not diabetic. So I enjoyed my lunch with a good helping of devilishly delicious desserts. By night, the hunger pangs were too cruel. On some days I would manage to get to my sleep despite the hunger. On the other days, I would give in.

There was something curious happening at this time. I was mortally hungry at night. But if I managed to get to my sleep, in the mornings, the hunger pangs were all gone! I would not feel tired even after a round of copious physical exercise. This was counter intuitive as by then I was farther away from my last meal. When I left sugar and sweets during the day, suddenly my hunger pangs in the night vanished! This was no less than a murder mystery for me!

Why does sugar make you feel hungry?

Sugar, in whichever form you take it, increases your blood glucose level immediately. When you take sugar, sweets or any high glycemic index food, there is a surge of glucose in the body- quite the reason why we feel a high when we take sugar. Our mood is elated.

The exact mechanism of insulin release in our body is something that doctors do not seem to agree upon. As an engineer trained in law, I find myself safe outside this debate. Some say that within a specified time, it is the same measure of insulin that is secreted irrespective of how much your eat. Some others say it is a proportionate relation between the amount of food eaten and insulin secretion. That is, more you eat, correspondingly higher amount of insulin amount of insulin is released. Or is it an asymptomatic exponential function? Let us leave that to the experts to debate and decide!

Anyway, when we take high glycemic index food like sugar, glucose level in blood shoots up. The issue being- anything that shoots up comes crashing down! So when the blood glucose level comes crashing down in while, we feel in extreme need of another shot of sugar. This cycle of snacking on the next sweet / high glycemic index food continues many times in the day. The number of times we eat food in a day rises. I once counted – mine was up to eight!

This surge and crash is typical of other psychotropic substances as well. But sugar does not get counted in this bracket (which I am concerned about). We are quick to suggest that there should be no advertisements promoting cigarettes and alcohol. But when it comes to sugary health drinks, we are not quite there in the level of awareness. The result is that about 400 million people are affected by diabetes on the planet. This leads to one complication or the other invariably – it might be kidney failure or loss of eye sight. Diabetes takes its toll.   And sugar is on a roll!

Apart from this surge and crash, that plays havoc with your day by making you feel low and dependent on other products like tea and coffee, sugar has one another issue with it. This is the highly concentrated amount of fructose in sugar. Fructose is naturally found in fruits. However, this is in a limited quantity and also clubbed with lots of fiber and other vitamins. When it comes to sugar, the fructose that would be found in quite a number of fruits, is concentrated and ingested in one go. The metabolism of fructose in liver is qualitatively different.

The technical details of this metabolism can be found in 'The Bitter Truth' by Dr. Robert Lusting. The video is again available on the Youtube. The crux of the matter is that fructose gets converted into fat which blocks our arteries and veins and renders us susceptible to heart attacks and strokes.

Now, that sugar is dangerous is not easy to appreciate! We live in an environment conditioned by advertisements, where one product after the other compete for our cognitive capture. Most of the food items in the super market have sugar in built in them. The movie 'That Sugar Film' clearly brings out the new jungle in which we are living in today. Sugar is out there on the prowl and pounces upon us from all corners.

It is a nice mental exercise to note how much of sugar comes our way every day. We are a society addicted to sugar. Our pleasantries and festivities are so infested with sugar that it is quite difficult for us to see what is right in front of our eyes.

When I make the unpopular suggestion of leaving sugar and sugar products, intellectual appreciation is almost immediate. But when it comes to avoiding sugar, I find the intellectuals getting physically stuck at what I call an attempt in moderating an addiction. They try to control the intake of sugar rather than completely avoiding it. One shot a day is bound to set you on the glucose surge–crash cycle which will make you feel terrible at the end of it. This is the reason why I give the same advice to you that my mother gave me about "drugs" when I was about to go to college – say no the first time. When it meets you the second time, you are weaker!

The social addiction to sugar and food in general is another difficulty. Our call-ons and conversations seem to be incomplete without a dash of sugar. When you look closely, you will find that the commerce involved is careful in developing and propagating this perception. #3SandOurHealth hopes to provide support in this regard by making a platform where we can discuss ideas on how to help save our relationships and lives from the commercial interests of a few.

In a way, the cruel thing about sugar is that it has now become so cheap that is has prevalence among the poorer people who cannot afford the negative effects of sugar. Look around yourself and you would find that with lesser financial resources, the diet tends to be more sugar intensive. Worse, the timing of sugar intake is also very random, this is exacerbated by the social addiction to sugar – making it mandatory in religious offerings and customary interactions. Sugar sticks!

CHAPTER THREE

AVOID SUPPER: HAVE YOUR LAST MEAL BY 1800 HRS.

Avoid supper: have your last meal by 1800 hrs.

Eating in the dark is so common in our society! So much so, that but for the Jain religion, there seems to be no other religion which even seems to suggest that one should finish one's last meal of the day before it is dark![1] However, if you speak to old people from the villages, they would tell you that eating after it is dark is something relatively new that has come into our society – at least in India!

It is easier to base such advice on the basis of religion. But my feeling is that, in the present generation, there is much more information flowing into us that if something is thinly anchored solely on religion, it would be deficient. So let us try to see why this suggestion of having an early last meal is being made.

Digestion slows down in the night – so says Dr. Suhas Kshirsagar says in his book 'Change your schedule, change your life'. It this be true, digesting anything ingested after dark would be a more laborious task. This task would not let our body rest properly. This is quite intuitive and I am sure all of us have experienced this when we have binged during dinner and then found ourselves uncomfortable going through our sleep.

When we have our dinner late, even though we seem to go to our sleep right afterwards, we are only getting an "eye-shut"-not sleep! The body cannot rest fully until the digestion process is over. So it is advised to complete the digestion work during our waking hours rather than trying to multitask during sleep.

In the same book, there is another interesting aspect mentioned regarding melatonin. Melatonin released into the blood stream is said to be helpful in repairing and cleaning up the body for the next day. But melatonin gets secreted only when the body believes that it is dark!

Dr. Kshirsagar very clearly brings out how watching screens of your mobile or the television during prime time deprives you of prime sleep! The full spectrum light will fox your body into believing that it is still day and so it would not release the required melatonin.

The delayed release of melatonin has the extra impact of making you feel groggy when you get up in the morning as the repair work is still going on! We often pressurize our kids to "get up early in the morning". After reading Dr Kshirsagar, I feel it is a misnomer that getting up at say 4 o'clock or 5 o'clock is termed as early. That is the right time to get up and one should be able to get up without alarm at this time. This can be achieved by laying emphasis on going to bed "early"- let me say, going to bed in time. This would in turn mean, getting ready to sleep early by giving the body a break from electronics after 6:00 p.m. Also the last meal for the day needs to be ingested before 6:00 p.m. This gives melatonin a full five –six hours to do its job by 3 AM in the morning.

This is easier said than done in the modern age without loss of efficiency and loss of socialization. Today our society has been so organised that we give maximum time to electronic screens and food at this critical hour of 7 to 10 p.m. What I would suggest is that you excuse yourself from asynchronous communication at this time and keep yourself available for synchronous communication! The last line is the electronics engineer in me coming back with vengeance. Let me clarify.

By asynchronous communication, I mean something like a WhatsApp chat where you do not have to be responding exactly at the same moment as the other person. Similar are social media platforms like Facebook or Twitter. If we keep these interactions for the morning, there is no great harm done.

A telephone call is a synchronous communication. It would require your immediate response. If you do not attend calls, you might be missing something really urgent and important. I have seen some keep a separate 'dumb phone' for this synchronous communication. That is not a dumb idea either! But this method would certainly not work with dumb bosses who would send you messages on whatsapp and expect you to reply instantly. This imagination that everyone lives online is very infective. I had a boss who would send something on whatsapp and when it is not "seen" in time, would send the reminder also on whatsapp!! No "S" can help them. May be "sense" can.

The most important reason why you should have your last meal by 6:00 p.m. is connected with insulin. When you have your last meal by 6:00 p.m, you get a full 12 hours before 6 a.m in the morning for the excess insulin to drain out of your body and for the body to reach a state of ketosis – a metabolic state in which body will burn fat for energy. This means that when you take your last meal by 6:00 p.m. your body is in a 'fat cutting mode' by next morning 6:00 a.m., when you could do your workouts. The fat loss during such a workout would be much more effective.

Insulin has two basic functions which it does whenever there is an excess of glucose in the blood stream. First, it starts converting excess glucose into glycogen thereby maintaining the blood glucose level. Second, it sends a message to fat cells not to burn. You would imagine that this is a sensible thing to do for the body. Since it has ready cash in the form of glucose, it is sending a message to the fixed fat deposit, not to get liquidated!

More the amount of fat we have in our body, more will be the insulin required for the second function of preventing fat burning. This would in turn mean that with more fat, your insulin release would tend to become less effective for glucose control. This is another name for diabetes! This also clearly brings out the link between obesity and diabetes, which is brought out in most medical text books.

When you have your last meal before six in the evening, by six in the morning, your body would have peacefully drained out the excess insulin and the fat cells would now be ready to be used up as fuel. This state of peacefully avoiding food can easily continue. As brought out in the last chapter, if one is avoiding the surge-crash cycle of glucose by avoiding high glycemic index food, then getting through to ketosis after the last glucose shot is easier. The body seamlessly shifts between using glucose as the fuel to using fat as a fuel. It won't be wrong to say that you feel hunger pangs because you take sugar!

Notes for the Chapter

[1]This is not correct. Recently I had been to Tokyo and was pleasantly surprised to note that they have the tradition of completing their meals before it is too dark. Many friends tell me that this was indeed the case in rural India before the breakfast-lunch-dinner paradigm got imposed on them. Come to think of it, even now, the Madhya Pradesh State Government offices starts functioning at 1030 hrs and closes by 1730 hrs – a relic of the earlier food habits in the region.

CHAPTER FOUR

AVOID MORNING TEA BEFORE WORKOUT.

Avoid morning tea before workout.

The mechanism explained in the last chapter is the reason why it is such a bad idea to have your morning tea before your morning exercise. Many of us do not have a well resting sleep during the night and so get up in the morning not feeling fully fresh. We then try to have a tea to 'get fresh'[1]. This releases insulin in our body which gives a message to the fat cells not to burn as glucose is around. The amount of glucose itself will be very less and will be fast depleted when one works out. But the insulin secretion ensures that burning of fat is no longer an option for the next twelve hours. This means that after the exercise, one is mortally tired and hungry. In this state, it is again natural for the person to take some instant energy foods which are sugars ! Ironically, most of our sugary energy drinks are positioned for exactly this occasion[2].

It is not unusual to find people sweating it out in the mornings without too much of an impact on their body fat. It is certainly not my case that exercise after morning tea is bad. It does have the other good effects of exercise like improving your blood circulation and releasing hormones like norepinephrine or endorphin. I am no expert in these and so would not elaborate more here. But it is certainly my case that if you are looking to lose that extra flab in your body and keep away from life style diseases, exercise during ketosis would take you to the ideal situation.

Exercise can be categorised according to its purpose-for reducing fat / weight, for improving stamina, for improving strength and for improving flexibility. All these four purposes are not all met by the same kind of exercise - so believe some experts. For example, if your intention and need is to lose weight, you should resort to aerobic exercises wherein you have rhythmic movements. This could be brisk walking, jogging or even swimming. But an exercise with jerky movements as in playing badminton or tennis would not be as helpful in losing weight. On the other hand, it would be helpful in building strength of your muscles. Stretching exercises like yoga would improve flexibility in the body. It is suggested that one should have a personal assessment of the needs of the body and do a good mix of exercises so that the above aims are achieved.

One should be cautious about taking the body to the appropriate weight before trying to suddenly jump on to the clay court after the French open. With more weight than necessary, it is quite possible that you will injure yourself in the attempt to play a sport. The first aim should be to bring your weight to the appropriate range. If you are aged below 50, you could try to gain on strength first and stamina thereafter. Post 50, it looks better to concentrate on maintaining the flexibility of the body by light exercises like yoga, while keeping your weight in check at the same time.

One word about stretching before your morning exercise is also critical here. This helps in preventing injuries. It would help you go on a for a longer duration which would be required to achieve your aims. Sports physicians lay special emphasis on stretching your calf muscles before you do a run. This simple investment of five minutes will go a long way in improving your schedule and your exercise.

Another question that is often asked is, about the timing of one's exercise- whether in the morning or in the evening? One would opine that exercising regularly has its own benefits because of the improved blood circulation and other factors. The improved blood circulation helps in removing toxins from our body.[3] However, if one has to choose a time, it would be mornings for the following reasons.

Typically, we are active in the day and exercising would be a way to prime us into this active state. An exposure to morning light would ensure that our body has a natural message that it is now morning and activity is expected. Dr. Suhas Kshirsagar brings out the connection with melatonin of this observed phenomenon. By having the body out in sunlight in the morning, it is a message that now melatonin can stop its work and let the body work.

When you are following the morning breakfast and late lunch schedule of intermittent fasting, body will be in a state of ketosis in the morning where you can achieve your goals from the exercise in a much better manner.

Initially when I started with intermittent fasting, I used to have products of refined sugar during my lunch in the form of desserts. After lunch, by dinner time, I would be mortally hungry. But ,if I braved this period of hunger and got to my sleep, I noticed that my energy levels were very good in the mornings. This was counter-intuitive as one was then farther from the last meal.

In a bout of inspiration of the movie "That Sugar Film", I left sugar. The impact on hunger pangs in the night was the most pronounced. Since there was no surge and crash of glucose levels, the avoiding of the evening meal was now much easier.

This again goes back to the importance of leaving sugar as given in the first chapter.

<u>Notes for the Chapter</u>

[1]Remember the advertisement of the new tea brand. You pull yourself out of the melatonin induced repair phase, complain that your body feels groggy and then give another externally induced reason for it to feel fresh!!

[2]Now you know the secret behind the secret of many celebrity sportsperson's energy (and bank balance)

[3]In Sanskrit, the term for exercise is Vyayam. Vyay is spending. Ama is toxin. Are we spending all our toxins in a regular manner or are we only accumulating them?

CHAPTER FIVE

AVOID SNACKS

Avoid snacks

Why should one avoid having small snacks after say every 2 hours? As on date, people are advised to be on such a diet by some leading dieticians to help in weight loss. I should state that some 5 years ago, I had also managed to lose some weight by going through this routine of having very small meals throughout the day. But my will power was not good enough to sustain this diet plan. In retrospect, I feel it was my luck that I did not stick to this plan which is not very sound in biochemistry.

To know why it is important to avoid snacks, we need to go a little deep into the biochemistry behind this. I strongly suggest watching the video by Dr. Jagannath Dixit in this regard. The mechanism is explained in short below-

In our body there is a basal level of insulin secretion by pancreas at all times. But whenever we ingest food and there is a release of glucose in blood level, a fresh bout of insulin is released in your blood. According to Dr. Dixit, this bout of insulin is not repeated within the next 55 minutes Presumably, this is the fill back time. If after 55 minutes, another trigger in the form of food is given, again another measure of insulin is released into the blood[1].

Now, one is still researching on the physiology of insulin release- on whether it is caused by ingestion of food or if it is caused by a higher remnant level of glucose in the body. Either way, repeated snacking will release insulin in the body which will have to send messages to fat cells also not to burn! This way, having multiple meals and not completing one's meal in 55 minutes would lead to an excess of insulin releases in the body[2].

Frequent releases of insulin leads to a situation of insulin tolerance[3]. That is, the effectiveness of insulin in the body goes down and the measure of insulin in the body would not be sufficient to keep the glucose level in check. This state is called diabetes in common parlance.

The long and short of the story is that snacking leads to diabetes. This can be measured by the rise in HbA1c level in the blood. This is an indication of the heightened blood glucose levels averaged over last three months. It later manifests as blood sugar. This heightened level of glucose in the body has deleterious effects on multiple organs. It is all too common to listen to gory stories of loss of eyesight or kidney failure in diabetes patients

<u>Notes for the Chapter</u>

[1] I researched to find out out about the physiology of the functioning of the pancreas. This claim of Dr. Dixit needs to be examined closely to see if it is indeed the case.

[2]This is typical of the late night parties where the first drink is brought to you at 7 PM and the desert is being indulged at 10 PM.

[3]Quite intuitive to Engineers. Just as we are unable to hear the ambient noise

16

CHAPTER SIX

MOVE TO LOW GLYCEMIC INDEX FOOD

Move to low glycemic index food

It cannot certainly be the case that instead of taking small meals after every 2 hours, one starts binging two three times a day. Moderation in food intake would certainly be necessary.

In this context, it is important for us to analyse what we are eating and how it affects our energy levels. This would also clarify why there is a suggestion for two square meals a day- what we used to pray for from our Gods[1].

When I used to eat my rice and dal or my roti and dal, I was not very sure if there was any purpose for dal-other than adding to the taste of the meal and giving the necessary protein. So I was rather unsuspecting when the new age life offered a bowl of pasta or noodles instead of my roti-dal-sabji combination. When one analyses food on the basis of glycemic index, the traditional diet suddenly stands out as the choice to be made. So does the practice of adding ghee to roti. I proceed to explain.

Glycemic index of food denotes the pace at which it releases glucose into the bloodstream. That is, a food item like potato with high glycemic index will release glucose all in one go like a sprinter. Food items like sprouts or milk with low glycemic index will release glucose slowly into bloodstream.

That is, when we eat our rice and dal, rice (being of higher glycemic index) releases glucose faster and dal (of lower glycemic index) follows suit a little later. This gives us stable energy levels for a longer time period. But when our meal is not square, all of the glucose gets released quickly. This glucose surge is a sudden bout of happiness for the brain as in the case of chocolates. However, in long term it is followed by a crash where the glucose levels come crashing down leaving us panting for more food.

This surge crash cycle is switching the power supply on and off in our body. This analogy would suggest that despite the feeling of happiness that high glycemic index food offers, we should make a conscious move towards low glycemic index foods.

When one looks at the spectrum of high and low glycemic index foods, it is quite revealing that what we know to be junk food are all high glycemic index items. We have a roaring snacking industry based on these food items. Poor *dal* does not have too many people packaging it, as it is not appealing to the surge and crash sensibilities of commerce!

This also suggests why we should move to square meals- first three and then two in a day. This will reduce the amount of insulin release into body and thereby ward off diabetes. But the two meals a day routine would be easy to maintain without debilitating hunger pangs. This happens only when you leave out the poison of sugar from your diet!

Notes for the chapter

[1]I heard an argument that two square meals was the bare minimum and that is why we included this in our prayers. The suggestion was that one should eat more frequently. For some reason, I have full faith that our God is quite capable of delivering what we pray for. If a third meal was necessary or preferable, our forefathers would have certainly asked for it. I can't remember myself holding back when I was praying for something from the Gods. I can't remember praying for the second rank in class as a kid!

CHAPTER SEVEN

NATUREATARIAN

Natureatarian

A note on 'natureatarian' is in order. When we are approaching food laid out in a buffet, all of it is equidistant from us. Be it a fruit, which has just been plucked from the tree or be it a processed piece of chocolate cake, which went through multiple layers of sophisticated handling to reach its present shape. When all food is equidistant, it is not immediately obvious to us that these foods have travelled different distances to reach us on the table that we are approaching.

The idea behind being a natureatrian is being aware of this aspect of food. Whenever we make a decision about what to eat and what not to eat, we should base our decision on a mental calculation of the distance travelled by the food from its naturally occurring state. Is it just out of nature? Or is it a broiler chicken which was farmed? Is it rice which is a product of cultivation or is it a nut which is just there in the nature? Is it a locally available food or is it an exotic and esoteric food which has been artificially collated to suggest that it is available in plenty?

This mental calculation will help us decide what is best to eat. To the extent we keep our food natural, we should be safe!

What do you have on your plate?

If there is one advantage of prime time TV, it is the identification of what commerce is pushing us to eat and drink. It may not be necessary for us to even know about these options. We would not have eaten these food items without the nudge, push, emotional blackmail and brainwash carried out through advertisments.

Thanks to the three Khans and their six packs, there is a heightened awareness and eagerness in the younger generation to eat healthy and to be healthier. In some cases, it does degenerate into quick fix solutions of deleterious protein packets. However, the new generation is much more health conscious than the cigarette smoking past.

When it comes to food, we have our own divisions. There are the vegetarians and non vegetarians. Then there are the lacto vegetarians and people who consider even onion, garlic and potatoes as taboo. We have godmen branding foods as *pranic* and *non pranic* – making one panic, by even including garlic in the *tamasic* category and sparing potatoes as *rajasvic*. Then there are nutritionists who insist that our grandmother knew best! If that be so, I should take to chewing tobacco!

The problem with food today, is that it comes to us on a platter! Let me explain. It is all too obvious in a buffet lunch or dinner. All these various tamasic and vegetarian and grand-motherian is accessible with the same amount of ease. The modern economy has put in economics of scale that brings the most esoteric item to the other corner of the world at a cost which is not helpful in making any distinction. So how do I choose what to eat?

The human body is like a machine which can convert energy in food articles and address its needs for locomotion. We have a relatively effective processor in our brain which is not very energy intensive. Perhaps, a perspective helpful in suggesting what food to take is to transpose our human body, by imagination, to the original environment it was designed for. i.e., before the 'artificial' intelligence of human beings started changing the circumstances (nature).

Here, I would not get into the debate if it was God who made this design. It is quite akin to the laptops and desktops we design with an expectation about the environment they would be in; and then suddenly, artificial intelligence takes over to change the environment itself without still being able to crack the code on how to change the power supply arrangement which was originally based on 230 V and 50 Hz.

So let us step back and give a thought – what are the natural foods available? How natural is a particular food item?. In today's buffet, the apple and the Chicken Muglai are both at the same level of effort. But in those days, for the hunter-gatherer, apple would have been a low hanging fruit (if you are in the right area) and chasing a fowl down would have been an engaging chase.

As the artificial intelligence of human beings have changed the backdrop, the natural stupidity has failed to distinguish between the different items on our plate. The level of physical activity that at least needs to follow taking different types of food are not obvious – given that there is no effort, whatsoever, preceding our access to these food items.

It would be helpful to mentally calculate the amount of processing and innovation that has been built into each food item. This would select a boiled egg over an omelette as the former is innocent of salt and oil – both 'secret' ingredients which make the omelette "highly processed"! We carry salt to distances where they could not have been thought of. We make oil available with no physical effort as a precursor. It is not to suggest that one should completely stop taking salt or oil given the processing involved. It is only a perspective which is suggested to see the food item as it is.

It is not rare to find vegetarians looking down upon non vegetarians as being unkind to kill a being to eat it. It is however lost on many of the veggies that even plants have life and pretty mute ones. For eating the cereals that we do, it is imperative that we farm them and terminate their lives to devour its seeds – all of it beaming with life, only seeking abandon to flourish. This argument is not to exculpate the non vegetarians. May be, we would not survive without this harvesting of mute lives. However, we need to be aware of our action even as we bite into our next *roti*, that the difference between vegetarians and non vegetarians is one of degree and not of kind – at least as far as the emotional side in concerned.

Again, looking at the "preceding effort perspective", helps us choose between the various types of vegetarian or non vegetarian food. You could picture your chances of being able to wrestle down a bovine. At least it does suggest to you that your body is designed to do more effort if it were to consume cereals rather than fruits or vegetables. This can only raise your physical activity given today's necessity of cereals for everyone to survive. If you can manage, change over to fruits (and that too local ones)!

We have a lifestyle in which we take pride in avoiding effort. This is not to discredit all the countless inventions and discoveries that help us live the lives that we do - and the technology that takes my thoughts to you. But, it is imperative for us to step back to see how much of the maze is our own creation, and play the game of life accordingly. The suggestion is to be listening to nature. It has more answers than the questions that we have managed to ask.

#natureatarian

CHAPTER EIGHT

WAY FORWARD

There are many diet systems like veganism, vegetarianism and Jain food habits which are considered to be more sattvic. As on date, I have not experimented with these. I strongly feel that these would certainly be much better as a food style and one should aspire to be following this. I am stopping at the suggestion of calibrating your *natureatarianism* for two reasons.

1. I am not qualified to suggest anything more, as I am not following that.
2. I do not find merit in taking the prescription too far away from the present state of the general population.

It should be doable and more importantly, felt to be doable. Everybody is different and what suits every body is different. So, I would encourage you to try out the elements mentioned in the book. It entails no extra expenditure. There is no fancy equipment or supplement that you need to buy. It is a safe deal!

I conclude with this word about sugar and the social addiction that surrounds it. My personal experience has been that moderated addiction is very sapping on your willpower. It is easier to say a complete no. It is so with alcohol. It is so with cigarettes. It is so with sugar! No apologies for the bracketing!

If at all my words have been able to give you a perspective, I will consider my work done. Everybody is different. One needs to be in touch with one's own mind, spirit and body as one charts the course to better health—weight loss, better sleep or better energy. The uniqueness of your body and spirit entails that you chart your own course after you listen to the logic expressed. I look forward to your word on the perspective. More selfish than most thoughts, since I am practising this, I need to know if I am making a mistake.

I repeat the 3S suggestion

Avoid 3S: Sugar, Snacks, Supper
Adopt 3S: Sports, Sangeet, Sleep.

I wish you luck and Godspeed!

CHAPTER NINE

MISCELLANEOUS

It would have caught your eye that the suggestions that I make in this book are quite in tune with what is prescribed in the traditional lifestyle of Indians. Ayurveda suggests the same as is brought out by Dr. Suhas Kshirsagar in his book.

This is sometimes a blessing as the base of the traditional way helps in adoption of a course by some. I believe I have been able to indicate some scientific reasoning to what is being suggested without leaving my argument to base itself only on tradition.

Especially when it comes to intermittent fasting, I believe there is always a possibility for the new generation to ask for more evidence than just tradition and a possible scientific explanation.

First, I would seek your indulgence in trying it out. In the Engineering colleges, this is the typical lure that is adopted to introduce the new generation to all sorts of deleterious activities- from smoking to drinking and more. Be that as it may , the challenge of an experience here is certainly not dangerous . After all, what am I asking for? Leaving sugar, eating one meal less, not watching mobile or TV after dark.None of this should kill you! If you derive benefits from that, go on.

But before you leave it, there is a need to know about some research that suggests about gains which may not be immediately obvious as it happens at a much deeper level. Here, I would like to refer you to the research of Doctor Yoshinori Ohsumi who got the Nobel Prize for medicine in 2016.

His research was about a process by which bodies feed on the dead cells and toxins in the absence of regular food after a period of fasting.

This suggests that if there is a period of fasting, it would be helpful in detoxifying our bodies.

In the Indian traditional system, we have the additional fast we observe during *Navratri*[1]. This typically happens just before change of seasons- at a time when people have a greater chance to fall sick. Is it a coincidence that a practice that detoxifies your body has been incorporated into our life by fixing it up into a religious calendar? It would have been very difficult to convince the masses about the biochemistry involved even if someone knew about it. But in an age where there is access to information, we need to do the hard-work of backing our suggestions with available evidence and openly acknowledging when we are unsure. The purpose of writing is not to pontificate. It is to document thoughts so that the next thought could start from where the earlier one ended! This book might have a copy right. But the idea is copyleft – seeking improvement or even rebuttal!

[1]Nine nights

CHAPTER TEN

Three S and our health: An IAS officer's guide to good health

"The Week"

Three S and our health: An IAS officer's guide to good health
September 27, 2019 22:41 IST

In a letter to an old friend, an IAS officer writes on the importance of avoiding sugar, snacks and supper and adopting sports, sangeet and sleep

Dear David,
How have you been? It's been a while since I wrote to you. The reason why I thought of rushing this letter is lest you have trouble in recognising me when we meet next! I am not joking—I have lost about 16kg since we last met. That is about how I look and weigh, but more important is about the positive change in how I feel.

With God's grace, I have a new routine where I am up and active early in the morning and am able to stay energetic all through the day. I have a rather punishing schedule, but my body, mind and spirit have only turned younger.

As you know, I have always wanted to be healthy, and I have been trying many diets and exercises. I have had some momentary successes, too—a fruit/vegetable diet gave me some relief from chronic sinusitis and having small meals every two hours, as suggested by some reputed dieticians, helped reduce my weight. All of it involved a lot of stress and use of willpower. But I have not been able to hold on to any of those. Now I feel that it was a blessing in disguise. I will tell you how.

I will try and maintain a bit of suspense. I will start by telling you what I went through. Today, I strongly believe that there is an easier path to the same result. But the comparative ease of the path I am suggesting is not immediately obvious if I do not speak about how I came to the conclusion.

It all started when I was still in Bhopal, about two years ago. I have a Maharashtrian friend in the service whose wife is a doctor. Hence, it was natural for discussions on health to come up in conversations. I got to know about the Dr Dixit diet plan from this family—a typical instance of education through WhatsApp university. The link that was shared was a video of Dr Jagannath Dixit, talking to what I understand to be medical students about a diet plan that is said to have been popularised by Dr Shrikant Jichkar (who is no more). The video stood out for one reason—it did not seem to be selling anything. In the video, which is available on YouTube, the key idea is this—have food two times a day; complete your meal within 55 minutes, avoid refined sugar and sweets if you are diabetic.

The logic is this: any act of having food will secrete a fixed measure of insulin in the body. Therefore, more the number of times you eat, more will be the measures of insulin released into your blood. More insulin in blood causes insulin tolerance. This, in turn, means more insulin would be required to deal with the same amount of glucose in blood. This, when not available naturally in the body leads to a dependence on externally administered insulin or drugs —a condition called diabetes. If a person eats food within 55 minutes, only one extra measure of insulin finds its way into blood and so insulin sensitivity of the body is maintained. A committed band of volunteers is now associated with Dr Dixit's mission of spreading awareness about this diet plan. It is claimed to even reverse the state of diabetes.

I decided to give this diet a try. By this time, I had relocated to Mussoorie and as you know my family could not move in with me. I know only to eat. No ideas of cooking were pursued after my debacle in some initial attempts in this regard. Getting three ready meals a day was a challenge, or perhaps the right environment where one was forced into the Dixit diet. I used to have my breakfast. I would have a late lunch. When I was not cheating Dr Dixit with a helping of muesli and flavoured milk in the night, I remained faithful to the diet by avoiding snacks.

The conditions in the Academy [Lal Bahadur Shastri National Academy of Administration] are helpful for maintaining health in some ways, but not in other ways. The academy had one of the best sports facilities on the planet. With my residence in the Happy Valley, I would have been hard-pressed for any excuse to not exercise. Again, there was the perceived moral responsibility of being a faculty who had to impress upon the trainees the need for physical fitness and discipline. So, being out in the morning to work out was easy.

On the flip side was the ready availability of snacks. My children used to adore my office. My little one was almost sure that her dad had the best of times alone in the hills with ready access to brownie and softy. The mess in the academy is blessed with the finest chefs who can test your willpower when you are trying to avoid snacks to adhere to Dr Dixit's plan. I used to virtually push all of these goodies into the 55 minutes at lunch time. Dr Dixit gives a license for 55 minutes; he never insists that we should eat for 55 minutes. But being faculty coordinator in law, I was quick to pounce on this loophole. I binged twice a day! But more often than not due to sheer nonavailability of dinner cooked at home, one tossed and turned into sleep to avoid the alternative of calling for another meal from the mess.

I lost weight. I would say I was exhausted with my consumption of willpower. I was reading about how willpower is available in a limited quantity, unlike brain power and muscle power which improve with usage.

But with regular exercise and a diet much more controlled than most others, I was losing weight. I kept reading about the advantages of intermittent fasting. It was a surprise to know about the Nobel Prize for medicine being given to Dr Yoshinori Ohsumi for his study on autophagy, which seemed to give a scientific basis for the religious practice of fasting.

I observed one thing here. After my lunch, by dinner time, I was hungry. But if I was able to get through to sleep, in the mornings there was no craving for food. I was not feeling as hungry or tired as on the previous night—not even after the five games of badminton in the mornings.

I then had an opportunity to go to South Korea. There was an invitation to be a resource person in a workshop on Disaster Resilience. You might remember that the last time I had been to Seoul, I had been smitten by the concept of Advaita philosophy having practical applications in everyday life. This time around, the message was quite simpler—quit sugar!

During a break in the workshop, I had a conversation with participants from the University of New Castle in Australia. When the topic of discussion came around to diets, one of them suggested that I watch *That Sugar Film* and sent me the link to the film. With some time available at my disposal, I watched the documentary. The gist of the film—how we are surrounded by the business of refined sugar and how social addiction to this is deleterious to the health of the society.

But why should one leave sugar? I strongly suggest that you watch the film to find out in detail. Robert Lustig, an American paediatric endocrinologist, has elaborated the biochemistry behind this in an academic manner and tried to elucidate the case. I try to state it here in layman's terms—sugar is fructose and glucose. Glucose is necessary for our body to cater to its energy needs. Glucose is received from carbohydrates, too, when they are processed. However, fructose is processed differently. If there is no immediate need for use, it is converted into fat inside the liver and it then gets deposited in areas where they can do most damage—like the blood vessels. So it is deleterious to take fructose in a concentrated manner, as in refined sugar or products that have a lot of refined sugar—from fruit juices to jams to ketchups. When we have sugar, it momentarily spikes our glucose levels and then when it comes down, it takes us into a dump where we feel low and crave for more sugar, much like any other psychotropic drugs! It would be better for our brain if the glucose level does not fluctuate so during the day. The brain works on glucose. So it would be beneficial to have our meals in the least number of times possible as this avoids the massive glucose swings all through the day.

Another key point here is the issue of burning deposited fat—a dream for many health aficionados. When we take food, the glucose supply goes up in blood and to help glucose unlock the cells for access, insulin is secreted. Now the suggestion is that insulin has another property, too. It sends a signal to the fat cells that they are not to burn. That is to say, fat won't burn when insulin is around. Once glucose in the body releases a measure of insulin, to drain it fully from the body to enable fat to burn, it requires twelve hours to elapse. So once you release your insulin with your morning tea, exercise will tire you down, but may not burn your fat. Here comes in the philosophy of intermittent fasting.

You would remember from the diet plan advised by Dr Dixit that one was to eat only two times a day and remain on water for the rest of the time. This and the age-old Jain tradition of having one's last meal before sunset helps in draining out the insulin fully from the body during our sleeping hours. Then when you do some bit of aerobic exercise in the morning, insulin is not around and the body turns into a mode of ketosis. This is a very good state— something I felt during my morning workouts in the academy. Since I was taking products of refined sugar during my lunch, I had a momentary high and then by evening my glucose level crashed and I felt I needed food. By morning, I was on ketosis if I braved through the crash, and I felt good.

This meant that if I left sugar, I should be able to do my two times a day Dixit diet in an easier manner and this is exactly what happened. I started losing my fat deposits and my weight started reducing. My energy level was very good as the glucose levels were stable rather than soaring up and crashing down. I was not releasing insulin every now and then, leading to insulin tolerance. I need to check my HbA1C levels to know how I am faring. This is considered to be a better measure to know how close to diabetes one is.

The best part was the depth of my sleep. With food in your belly, even when one closes one's eyes, the body is still working and has little time to really rest and recuperate. This means that even with a longer sleep, the depth required is not available, Avoiding mobiles and TV before sleep spares you from a visual stimulus overload and contributes to the third dimension of your sleep. I was having better sleep.

I have thus come to the philosophy of 3S and our health. I say adopt 3S and avoid 3S. The 3S to be avoided are sugar, snacks and supper, in that order. The 3S that is to be adopted would include sports, sangeet (music) and sleep.

As remarked earlier, willpower is limited. So, even if we embark on a journey with willpower, we should soon seek to load it on to some other source of power—the power of routine. To lose weight, if we get into a routine where it would then require willpower to break away from might be the best course.

I will close with one observation I could make when I quit sugar in South Korea. Suddenly I was looking for food in the supermarkets without sugar. It was an eyeopener that I could not find anything but peanuts. The sugar movie says 80 per cent of what we eat has sugar. The limit of sugar consumption for human safety advised by benevolent medical associations is seven teaspoons and we are consuming more than 30. Just one bottle of soft drink has around seven teaspoons! I feel that it is easier to personally come out of the poisonous sugar consumption, but to bring out one's family, friends and the society is quite another struggle. The commerce involved is certainly not helping. There is a whole industry built around burning of excess calories, which also happily coexists with the commerce of refined sugar. Not to speak of the medical industry that tries to prevent the millions of death caused by diabetes!

It is time that we disbelieve that any boost is the secret behind someone's energy. We need to look for our own secret to boost our energy—avoid sugar, snacks & supper, and adopt sports, sangeet and sleep.

CHAPTER ELEVEN

ADOPT 3S MANTRA FOR GOOD HEALTH

"The Pioneer"

Adopt 3S mantra for good health
Saturday, 12 October 2019 |

There is a need for concerted action to educate people about the deleterious effects of refined sugar and sweet products

The demands of modern society put a strain on the lives of almost everyone on the planet — not just bureaucrats or babus as they are known in the country. Though the work-related stress that babus undergo is particularly bad, given their responsibilities, I am quite accommodative of the suggestion that all of us are in it together. We all face the stresses of everyday life, the yearning for good health and the dread of lifestyle diseases. These considerations led me on a quest for a healthier lifestyle and a fitter, leaner body. Consequently, two years on, I am 16 kilograms lighter. I have started rising early. And, despite having a punishing work schedule, I feel active and am able to channelise my energy more productively throughout the day. I even sleep better now.

However, the journey to this state of bliss and well-being was not easy. It started two years ago while I was in Bhopal. A friend's wife, who was a doctor, introduced me to Dr Dixit's diet plan on YouTube. To me, the credibility of the video was mostly because it was not trying to sell anything. The plan involved eating two meals a day, finishing a meal within 55 minutes and avoiding refined sugar, particularly if one was suffering from diabetes. The biochemical reasoning offered was simple — every time you eat, insulin is released. This, in excess, leads to insulin resistance and diabetes.

I opted for this diet when I relocated to Mussoorie at the Lal Bahadur Shastri National Academy of Administration. Without my family around and with no experience in the kitchen, it was easier to skip dinner. As I was not diabetic, I continued to have sugar and sweet products during the two "binge windows" in the day. Though I felt mortally hungry at night, somehow I managed to get through that phase.

With a healthy dose of exercise and the diet plan, I lost weight. There were times when I nearly lost my willpower, and matters were certainly not helped by the queer circumstances which kept my family away in Bhopal. Though getting to sleep without dinner was a massive effort initially, by the time it was morning, there was no craving for food and one could relish the many games of badminton and squash in the beautiful Happy Valley. This was counter-intuitive for me, as by morning one was further away from the last full meal that one had eaten.

At this juncture, on the suggestion of a friend from Australia, I watched *That Sugar Film*, a movie that reveals all about the business of refined sugar and how "social addiction" to it is deleterious to health of the whole of society. This movie, which is in fact a well made documentary, was life changing.

When I use the word "social addiction" I want to indicate that it is not just the individual but the whole world which is hooked to this dangerous food, sugar. The movie prompted me to give up sugar and then I observed that the hunger pangs which used to bring me down at night completely disappeared. So what was happening? Let me explain.

Sugar (or any high glycemic index food) sends glucose levels soaring in the blood only to crash later on. When glucose levels dip, we begin to crave more sugar. This meant that if I cut sugar out of my diet totally, I would be able to follow my "two meals a day" Dixit diet easily. And, this is exactly what happened.

If you afford 12 hours for insulin to drain out of your body, the process of ketosis (when the body does not have enough glucose for energy, it burns stored fats instead; this results in a build-up of acids called ketones within the body) begins. I started losing my fat deposits and my weight started reducing. My energy level was very good as glucose levels were stable rather than soaring up and crashing down. The sports activities in the morning were now direct attacks on fat deposits. There was another happy outcome of this. Since the digestion process was well over by the time one retired for the day, sleep was undisturbed and complete, in the same number of hours as before.

There is a need for a concerted action to educate the next and the present generation about the deleterious effects of refined sugar and sugary products. The commerce of sugar, fitness and treatments stands at a risk with this realisation in the masses and so it should not surprise you if these words do not ever reach you in time. To sum it up, an immediate necessity for us is to "avoid 3S and adopt 3S," which means avoid sugar, snacks and supper. Adopt sports, sangeet (music) and sleep. The journey could be easier for you if you start by avoiding sugar. Then watch the 3S effect.

(The writer is an Indian Administrative Service officer of the Madhya Pradesh cadre. The views expressed are personal.)

CHAPTER TWELVE

TEA OFF YOUR DAY!

Tea off your day!

Raghuraj Rajendran

Lodhi garden in Delhi is a beautiful place to be at 6'clock in the morning! So are the other little and big parks in the cities where the health conscious elite gather to participate in the Fit India campaign by having their morning dose of sporting activity.

I suspect that most of the enthusiastic lot who get to these sports activities are not very satisfied with the results. Yes, the morning walk is refreshing; but the fat deposits seem to be stubborn – One gentleman quipped- Pran Jaye, Par Wajan na Jaye! (I am dying, but my weight is not going away). Without the body being in proper shape, many come back bruised after they endeavour to exercise with new found enthusiasm!

There are one or two simple things that you could try to get better result out of your morning sports.

First, avoid tea or any insulin stimulating drink or bite before your morning activity!

'Why? That gives me the energy to get on with my morning?!'

Let me elaborate! When you have tea, with sugar OR milk, before your exercise in the morning, there is all probability that you trigger an insulin release in your body. Insulin has two roles. It converts excess glucose to glycogen. But it also sends a signal to fat cells not to burn - now that glucose is available!

So, having your morning tea means that your body which was about to get into state of ketosis after the overnight fast, gets back to being on glucose. Fat lives on for another day!

It you leave out that morning spike of insulin, your morning activity will cut down your fat deposits. This will improve your ability to stretch yourself more with sports activities as you move towards your ideal weight.

Again, when you exercise be clear about your reason to exercise. If you are overweight, are you trying to cut out fat and reduce weight? Or are you trying to improve your flexibility? Or are you trying for muscle strength? This is important is as your aim will determine the kind of exercise that is best for you.

For weight loss, it has to be aerobic exercise, says some experts. For muscle strength, it ought to be anaerobic exercise. You would know many amateur badminton players who sweat out their three games on the court along with their pot belly fully in place for years! To burn away your belly, you need to reach that state of ketosis where insulin spikes are not blocking it. Aerobic exercise like brisk walks or jogging would be required. It would be important for you to first get in proper shape by reducing your weight (if you are overweight) before you jump out into that court for your game of badminton.

Now to reach a state of ketosis at 6 a.m. in the morning, apart from avoiding your morning tea before exercise, you need to do your body another favour- don't put in food into it at night when it is not at its best in digestion! A basal level of insulin secretion is a given; but to get the body rid of the excess insulin, the body must be given a break of about 12 hours. So, having your food before 6 PM in the evening will give that critical time for your body, when you can hope to cut down on your fat deposits. It is quite like the body telling you that you have to spend the ready cash in hand before you dive into the fixed deposits. It is only being logical!

Now, if you manage to have an early last meal of the day, it also helps you in getting better sleep. Your body is not having to do digestion when you are having your eyeshut (distinguishing it from a rejuvenating repairing sleep). Here again, the spectrum of light from the screens – mobile or TV tells us our body that it is day when it is still night at nine in the night. This delays the secretion of melatonin, which repairs our body and gives us rest. This rest is as critical to be able to get up fresh early in the morning. But alas! We have always tried to get up early in the morning forcing our way out of bed to be good boys and girls and felt groggy in the morning in the bargain! It was 'Early to bed and so Early to rise' – but we seemed to miss the point. Prime time TV OR Prime time sleep – sorry about that !

Getting out in the sunlight will give our body the necessary message to keep it lively. This is true at 6 AM in the morning and so it is at 4 PM in the evening. So the sun might help us to take the Tea (and the sugar) out of our day. Then we will Tee off our day!

The author is a member of the Indian Administrative Service of the Madhya Pradesh cadre. The author can be reached at raghurajmr@gmail.com. The views are personal
#3SandOurHealth

References And Notes

1. Effortless Weight Loss and Diabetes Prevention by Dr. Jagannath Dixit
2. Change your schedule, Change your life by Dr. Suhas Kshirsagar
3. FAT chance by Dr. Robert Lustig
4. Pure, white and Deadly by Dr. John Yudkin
5. That Sugar Film by Damon Gameau